Energize

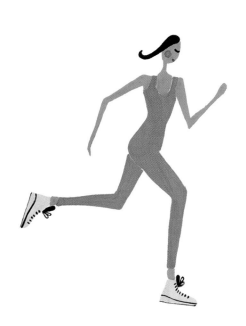

Energize

100 natural ways to recharge

Carol Morley & Liz Wilde

Time Warner Books

WARNER BOOKS

An AOL Time Warner Company

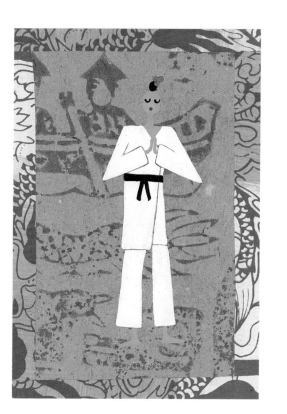

introduction

Are you tired all the time? Do you regularly have low-energy days when even the thought of getting out of bed makes you feel exhausted? Poor energy levels can be due to stress, diet, and even boredom. Stress sends an adrenaline rush through your body that uses up precious energy needed to keep the rest of you going. The food you eat supplies your body with energy, but if you're not eating enough of the right stuff, you won't have sufficient fuel to help you last through the day. And if you're stuck in a rut and bored with life, your mind (quickly followed by your body) will kick back and start working part-time. Understand what's sapping your energy levels and you can make a serious difference to your life. Just small changes will leave you re-energized and ready to go. This little book tells you how.

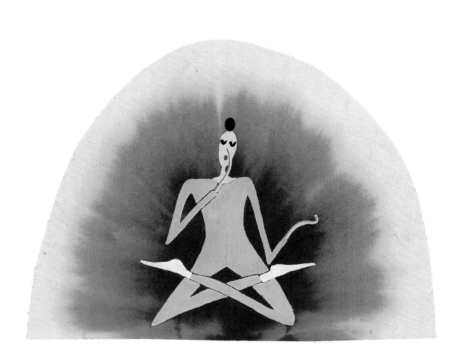

contents

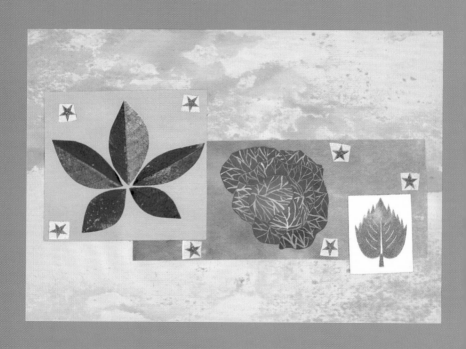

chapter 1

Eating for energy

1 **Carbohydrates are the best energy foods as they release sugar slowly into your bloodstream.** For a quick fix, eat whole-wheat bread, rice, and dried fruit like raisins and apricots. For a slow steady burn, choose complex carbohydrates like oatmeal, pasta, potatoes, and muesli. But steer clear of starches such as white pasta, bread, and rice, as these will send you off to sleep.

2 **Choose foods containing nutrients that allow your body to convert food into energy.**

Vitamin B—avocado, tuna, yogurt, chicken, eggs

Vitamin C—broccoli, Brussels sprouts, citrus fruit, green peppers, tomatoes

Vitamin E—asparagus, mangoes, brazil nuts, sunflower seeds, spinach

Iron—eggs, meat, shellfish, cereal, chickpeas, dried fruit

Magnesium—spinach, broccoli, grapefruit, apples, cashew nuts

Potassium—potatoes, raisins, pistachios, sunflower seeds

Zinc—brown rice, seaweed, pumpkin seeds, cashew nuts.

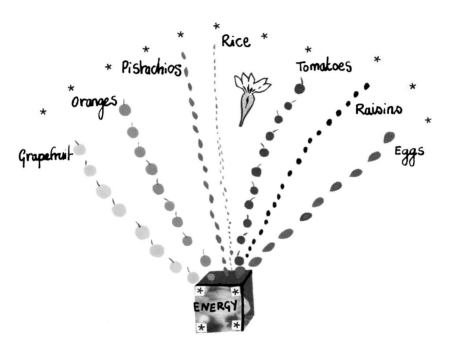

3 **When stress is sapping your energy, counteract the attack with plenty of energy-giving foods.** Fill up on food in its natural state, such as raw fruit and vegetables, whole-wheat bread, nuts, and seeds.

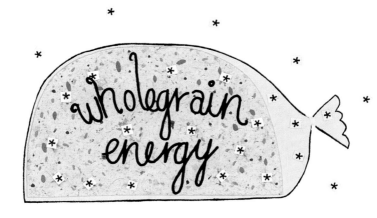

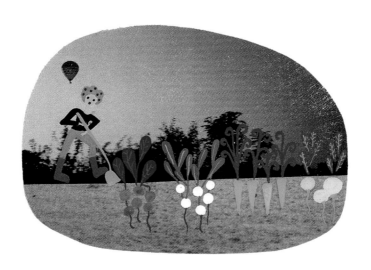

14

Eating for energy in a nutshell:

| Natural whole foods | = *energy givers* |

| Fatty, refined, and highly processed foods | = *energy sappers* |

Make every mouthful something that gives you energy, not takes it away.

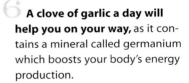 **In-Flight Energy Foods:**

- *Dried fruit (mangoes, dates, figs)*
- *Nuts (almonds, pistachios, walnuts, cashews)*
- *Bananas*
- *Bottled water (have a glass every hour you're airborne).*

A clove of garlic a day will help you on your way, as it contains a mineral called germanium which boosts your body's energy production.

7 Foods most likely to fuel you are plant-based, so fill your refrigerator with fresh fruit and vegetables. Green leafy vegetables contain vitamins C and E, beta-carotene, zinc, and iron—all nutrients that energize your body and brain. Make energy-packed raw juices like carrot and beetroot to get you buzzing. Buy whole-wheat bread and pasta, and brown rice. And choose the choicer cut of meat (i.e. lean and low fat) or fill up on fish. Vegetarian? No problem. Let beans be your protein punch.

8 Bouncing blood sugar plays havoc with your energy levels. Heavy meals make your energies dip, so stay stable by eating three light meals a day with healthy snacks in between. For a sweet fix, eat seedless white grapes rather than caffeine-packed chocolate.

9 Food gives your body energy, but not before taking some away during digestion, which is why you feel so tired after too much munching. Choose foods that break down fast—raw fruit and vegetables, nuts and seeds, brown rice, tofu, and virgin olive oils. In second place comes whole-wheat bread, chicken, fish, and goat milk. Heavyweight foods include red meat (which takes two days to digest), white bread and rice, microwaved food, sugar, and cow's milk dairy products.

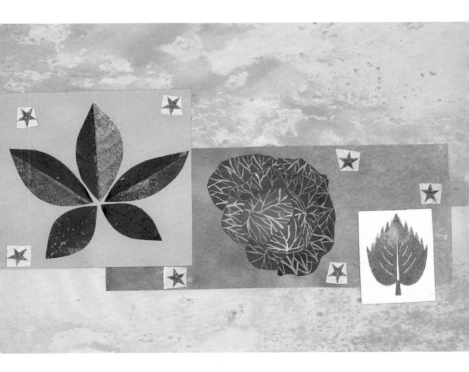

10 **Drop the diet.** Food provides your body with energy and the less you eat, the less you'll have. Calories are the energy we need to lead a healthy life, but the trick is to match the amount of calories you eat with the amount you burn up. Even when relaxing, your body is busy working, and if you're concentrating, all the better (the average brain uses about one calorie every four minutes). Very light work such as cooking burns between 80–100 calories an hour, moderate exercise like housework burns between 110–160, and more serious exercise, such as cycling or fast walking, an impressive 170–240.

11 **Bananas are the ultimate feel-good food.** They're rich in fiber and starch for quick-release, slow-acting energy, and also contain mood-enhancing ingredients like vitamin B6 and tryptophan—much better than a bar of chocolate.

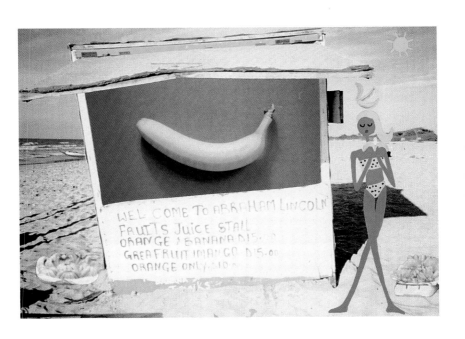

12 Feeling tired may be a sign that you're just dehydrated. Water is essential to the energy production going on in the cells of your body. Gulping two glasses of water will wake you up in minutes, and the faster you drink, the bigger energy surge you'll feel.

13 Coffee addicts should switch to decaffeinated beans, but beware the types of processes used to make them that way. Some involve using similar solvents to those found in paint strippers and dry-cleaning solu-tions. The coffee is then steamed to bring the beans' chemical level down to legal limits, but residues can remain. Play safe by choosing coffee decaffeinated with a water-only process—read the small print before buying.

14 For a healthy hot-drink high, try sipping rosehip tea, which gives you energy without the caffeine payoff later. Or make your own energizing ginger tea by grating a spoonful of fresh ginger into your hand and squeezing it into hot water.

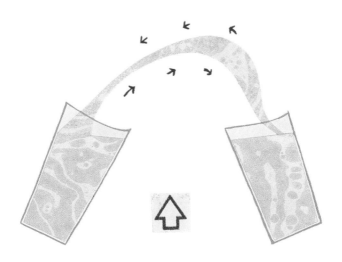

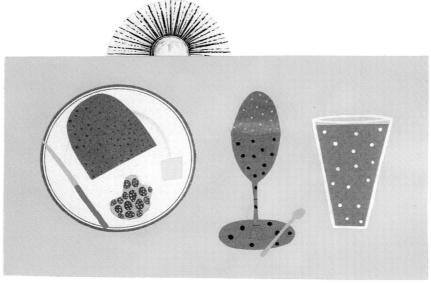

15 **What you eat (or don't eat) for breakfast determines how much energy you'll have for the rest of the day.** A cup of coffee simply won't cut it. What you need is a real meal that includes carbohydrates, protein, and fat. Eat a carbo-charged breakfast (plain toast, muffin, or bagel) and your energy will last for a couple of hours. Add slower-burning protein and fat to your plate, and you'll be buzzing all morning. More substantial breakfasts include whole-grain toast and peanut butter, poached or scrambled eggs on toast, or a wholewheat bagel and smoked salmon. Or try the model's favorite—a bowl of oatmeal. This complex carbohydrate releases energy slowly all day, making it perfect for when you're too busy for lunch. Not a morning person? Then it's even more important to find time for a breakfast fix.

16 The oilier the fish, the more omega-3 fatty acids it contains. These workaholics transport oxygen, remove cholesterol, lower blood pressure, and support the nervous system to help the body cope with stress better. And if this wasn't enough, fatty fish also raises energy levels by boosting your heart and circulation.

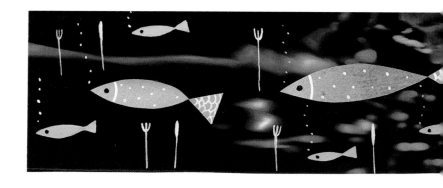

17 **Treat yourself to a Japanese meal at the end of an exhausting day.** Seaweed is known to boost energy levels, and a bowl of miso soup plus a seaweed salad will ensure you leave the restaurant with more bounce than when you went in.

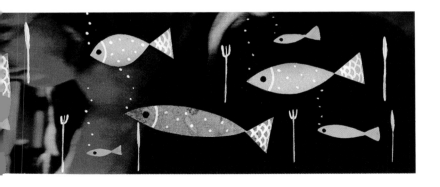

18 **If you're suffering from a serious energy slump** (and you're not sick), a nutritionist will know where you're going wrong. By checking which nutrients you're lacking, an expert can prescribe an eating plan to get you back into shape.

19 **When you've overeaten, your body has to clear the clutter, which takes more energy than usual.** A mini-fast could be just what your body needs to give it a break. Try eating only raw fresh fruit and vegetables for a whole day after overindulging. Drink plenty of water to help your body with the elimination process. Be aware that the more toxins there are in your body, the worse you're going to feel. Take it easy and plan a relaxing day while your insides are hard at work.

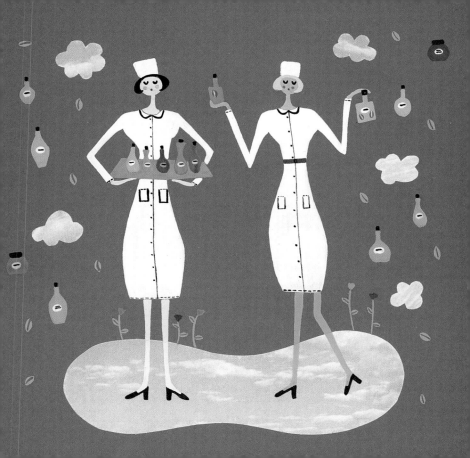

20 **Seeds and grains are packed with energy-giving goodness.** Buy bags in your local supermarket and grow your own. Soak seeds overnight, line a tray with nylon mesh to encourage drainage, and pour them in. Place the seeds or beans in a warm dark spot for three days. Spray them twice a day with water, then transfer them to a sunny spot for a few hours before eating them.

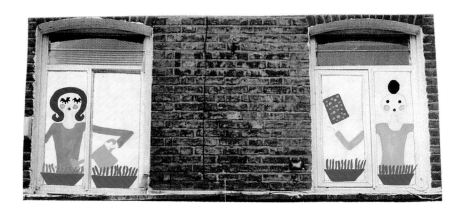

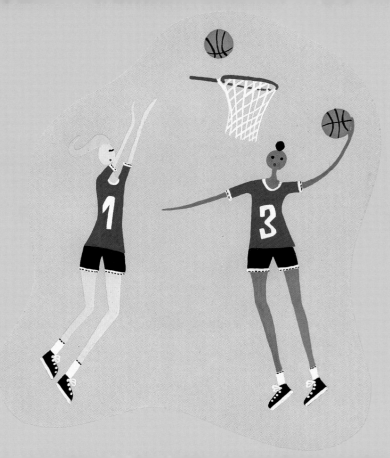

chapter 2

Exercise high

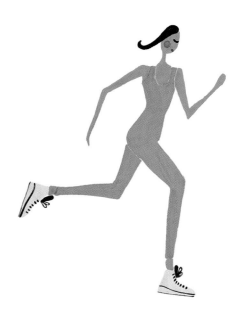

32

21 **Exercise regularly and you'll have more energy. That's a fact.** In recent studies, women who had never lifted a weight in their lives and started to keep fit suddenly had almost 30% more energy than ever before. But what if you don't have the energy to start exercising in the first place? Begin slowly and remember, any amount of activity makes you feel better than lying around on the sofa.

Need more convincing? Shock statistic: Researchers say that failing to exercise can be as harmful to your health as smoking a half pack of cigarettes a day. Now that's what we call an incentive.

22 **Heard of a runner's high?** Well, it's true. After a heart-pumping run, you'll feel you can take on the world. That's because exercise stimulates the body's pituitary gland which releases those feel-good endorphins. Research shows it's almost impossible to feel bad about yourself after a workout. Just don't sign up for that marathon until you've come down to earth.

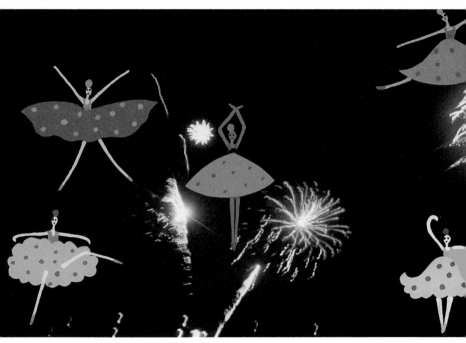

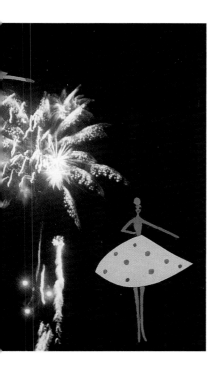

23 **Whatever you're doing, if you're fit, you'll be able to do it better.** That means dancing, gardening, sex, and even shopping, because exercise improves your stamina. They'll have to drag you off the dance floor.

24 **Modern fitness no longer means grueling hours spent at the gym.** Just thirty minutes, three times a week, of any activity that gets your body breathing harder than normal will raise your energy levels, relieve depression, oh, and give you the body you've always dreamed of.

25 **Walking is the best energy-fix around.** It not only increases your intake of oxygen and boosts your immune system, but also stimulates a tired body and mind. Walk briskly for at least 30 minutes, or make that an hour and you'll be happy to know you've also burned off around 400 calories.

26 **Always feel lethargic after lunch?** Then head outdoors for a ten-minute walk. Studies show this boosts energy for up to two hours after your stroll.

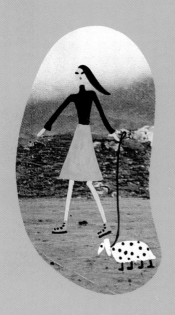

27 **Nowadays it's easier to send an e-mail than walk to another office for a chat.** We all know we should be active, but fewer than half of us are. So tear yourself away from your screen once in a while and go visit your friend on the fifth floor. If your boss catches you, blame it on a computer break —you're legally entitled.

28 **Another link between energy and exercise:** you can't feel energetic without the right foods to fuel you, and regular activity improves your body's ability to break down food by raising the oxygen levels in your bloodstream and increasing the efficiency of your heart.

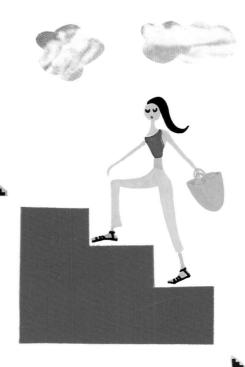

29 Weight training's not just for meat heads. A stronger body equals more energy. Why? The weaker you are, the more energy you need to keep going. So build more muscle and life will be a breeze.

30 When you've been ill, your body needs to rest and repair. But vegging out in the house for days and days will leave you weak and even more vulnerable to illness. Once you start to become better, the longer you stay on your sick bed (or sofa), the more tired you'll feel. But beware sudden activity which will leave you exhausted. Take it gently. Any new exercise routine needs to be done for at least a week before your muscles get used to the shock, then you can crank up the pace.

31 Even a gentle stretch can improve your energy levels and also helps calm a stressed-out mind. Stretching expands your chest area, giving your inner organs more room to operate. The result? Increased blood flow and more energy-giving oxygen rushing around inside you. Just a few minutes a day will do the job.

1. Stand up straight with your feet hip width apart and your fingers interlocked behind your head.

2. Take a deep breath in and, as you breathe out, push your arms up with palms facing upward. At the same time, feel your whole body stretching toward the ceiling.

3. Relax and repeat until you feel loose and lengthened.

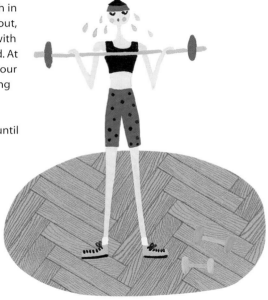

32 Exercising in the fresh air clears your head and inspires your mind. Cycling in the great outdoors is far more interesting than watching a row of gym-bound bikers, and outdoor exercise works you harder too. Consider the difference between a stationary bike in the gym and the open road. You're guaranteed to burn more calories as you power your bike up hills, around corners, and into the wind. It's far more energetic than reading a magazine propped up on the handlebars as you pedal.

33 You're never going to feel full of beans if you're feeling blue, but studies prove that regular exercise beats depression. Just four weeks of activity can seriously improve your mood. Guaranteed.

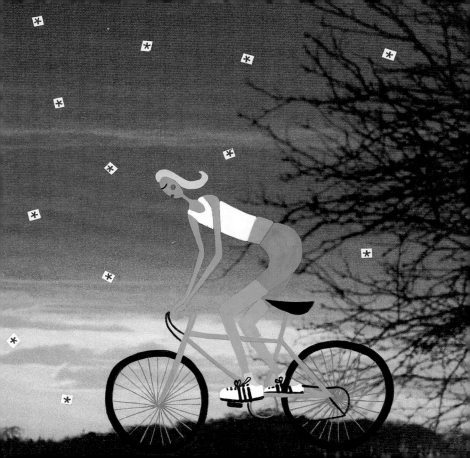

34 You know regular exercise makes you feel better, but you keep pushing that snooze button in the mornings until it's too late for anything more than a shower. It's hard to keep yourself motivated when exercising alone, but become part of a team and you'll find it tough to say no. Choose something you enjoy—basketball, football, tennis, a running club— and let your fellow exercisers inspire you. And don't worry if they're all so much more skilled than you. Do what you can and you'll soon catch up with the rest of them.

35 OK, so exercise can give you energy, but heading for the gym straight after a long tiring day will just make you feel worse. Instead, go home and get a good night's sleep and save your exercising for the next morning. And remember, vigorous exercise too late at night will stimulate your mind and body, making it harder to fall asleep later.

36 Don't be tempted to spend Saturday making up for your lack of exercise all week. A sudden burst of activity will leave you feeling exhausted, not energized. Instead, work exercise into the week, even if you're only walking to the bus stop and back. As with most things, little and often is better than all or nothing.

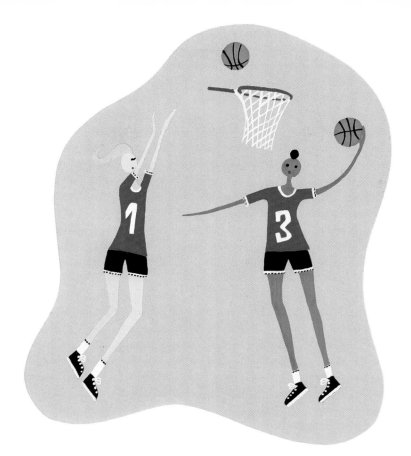

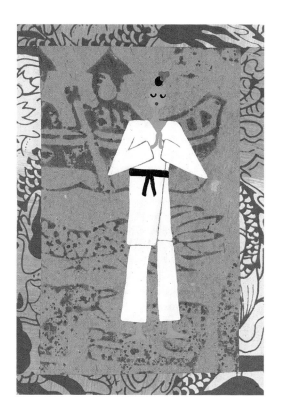

37 Ancient martial arts are the very latest way to get fit. Expect gentle movements in tai chi and qigong where the emphasis is on internal strength and a calmer mind. More physical by far are karate and judo—you'll learn a serious method of self defense while getting a great workout. Whatever you choose, all martial arts aim to energize the mind and body, sharpen reflexes, improve coordination, and promote mental relaxation.

38 Exercise doesn't just give your body energy— it energizes your mind too. Research has found that regular activity three times a week improves memory and judgment by 25%.

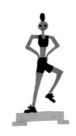

try anything from power yoga, Pilates, kickboxing, spinning to boot camp (pretending you're in the army). First timers should look for classes with the magic word beginner or basic in the title, and

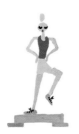

39 Are you allergic to aerobics? Gym classes have come a long way since legwarmer-wearing instructors high-kicked along to 1980s disco tunes. Now you can

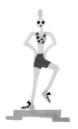

go along with a friend if shy. Just remember to keep your eye on the teacher and, if you lose the plot, march on the spot rather than stop dead in your tracks. Like any skill, expect to take

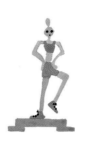

40 **For the maximum heart-pumping, fat-burning high, vary the intensity of your work-out** (known in the trade as interval training). A heart that goes up and down is working far harder than one that stays on the same level.

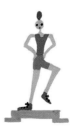

a few lessons to learn the ropes, and for the ultimate energy high, pick an instructor who shares your musical tastes. After 30 minutes of feel-good tunes, you'll be flying.

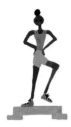

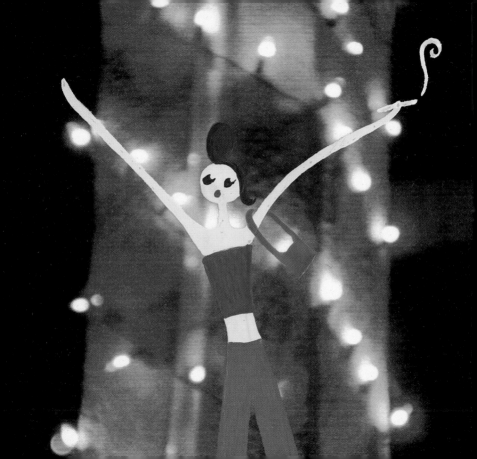

chapter 3

Energy enemies

41 Couch-potato pursuits like watching TV will leave you more tired then ever. Lying in front of the television all night is never going to fill you with energy. When was the last time you turned off the TV and jumped up, ready for anything? Chances are, by the end of the night, you've hardly got the energy to hunt for the remote control.

42 Work, home, bills, shopping, family commitments. No wonder adults don't have nearly as much energy as children. You may not be able to avoid the responsibilities of being a grown-up, but you can still find time to play like a child. Taking life too seriously will definitely sap your energy.

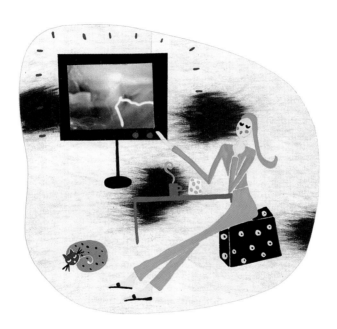

43 **Coffee and other caffeinated drinks (think hot chocolate, cola, and tea), give you an instant high, quickly followed by a low,** made much worse if you were tired in the first place. Drinking coffee to boost your energy will just set you off on a downward spiral, so stick to three cups a day, max. For every one you down, drink twice as much water to make up for it (caffeine is also a diuretic), or switch to tea, which gives a more subtle rollercoaster ride.

44 **Sugar works in the same way, shooting straight into your bloodstream.** The result? Your blood sugar level rises too rapidly, making your body race to lower it again. Expect an energy slump between one to three hours after tucking into a sugary snack.

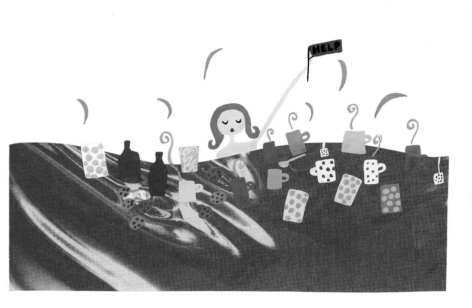

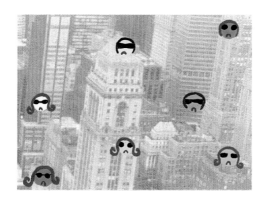

45 **A walk by the sea or in the country leaves you buzzing with energy. Why?** Because fresh air is charged with negative ions which stimulate the oxygenation of the blood and energize your body. No surprises then, that you feel your lowest surrounded by car fumes, electrical equipment, synthetic materials (i.e. carpets, curtains, and a cheaply covered sofa), cigarette smoke, and air conditioning, all of which reduce the level of negative ions present—another excuse to escape to somewhere green for the weekend.

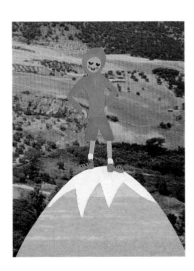

46 **Step out the front door and your body is bombarded with toxins.** These all put pressure on your immune system to work overtime, resulting in less energy for the rest of you. Do yourself a favor and don't add to the toxic overload by smoking. Inhaling cigarette smoke (even through passive smoking) exposes you to over 200 chemicals each time you (or someone else) lights up. Smoking also deprives your body of energy-giving oxygen and constricts your blood vessels, slowing your circulation and making your heart work twice as fast to compensate. Stop smoking now and experience an energy boost almost immediately.

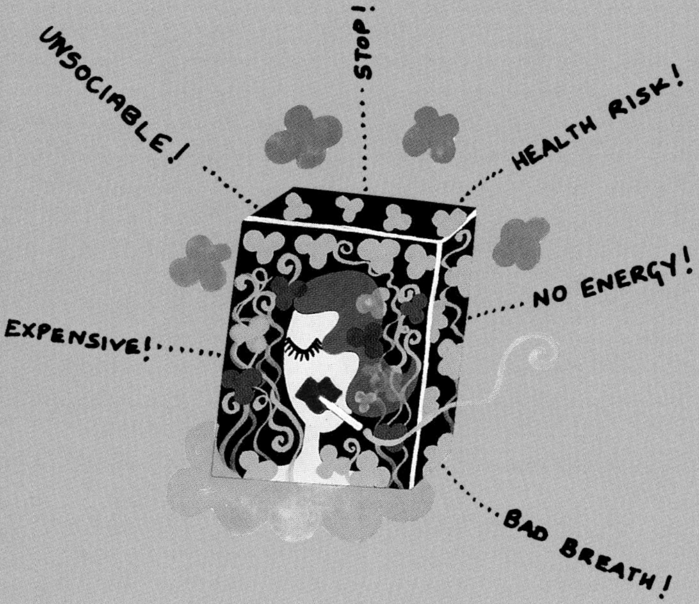
UNSOCIABLE!
STOP!
HEALTH RISK!
NO ENERGY!
EXPENSIVE!
BAD BREATH!

47 **When your stress levels are sky high, your body suffers an adrenaline rush,** which releases fatty acids and glucose into your bloodstream. As these are your body's main energy supply, a change in circulation will leave you feeling low. Some stress is good for motivation, but severe stress carries a serious health warning. Much stress is within your control. Identify what (or who) drives you crazy and plan how to cut it (or them) out of your life.

48 **Boredom drains your energy far more than being busy doing things you enjoy.** If you're stuck in a rut, climb out. A lack of new challenges will leave you lazy and apathetic.

49 **Many of us spend the day under outdated fluorescent lighting** which was originally designed to be a cheap, short-term way to extend working hours in times of darkness. Scientists have discovered that people who spend most of their time away from natural light suffer fatigue, headaches, and depression. Swap your lighting to full-spectrum bulbs (which simulate natural daylight), or go outdoors as often as you can for an instant lift. Artificial light actually suppresses the production of a hormone called melatonin. In animals it is responsible for hibernation patterns, so no wonder a day under flourescent lights leaves you feeling lethargic.

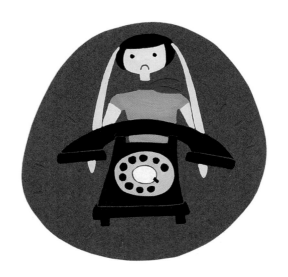

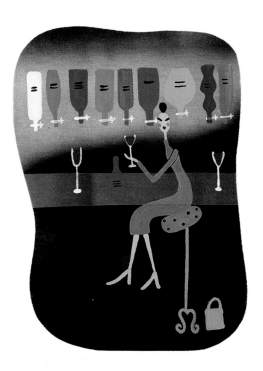

62

50 **When you're tired and low, you may feel the only way to get through the evening is with a permanent glass of wine in your hand.** But alcohol is a depressant. Sure, it may not feel like that at first, but wait until the alcohol hits your brain (about 20% gets there in seconds). It slows down both your movement and your mind. Not to mention the morning-after come-down. No one feels full of energy with a hangover.

51 **One or two glasses of wine can calm you down after a bad day**, but any more will stop you sleeping soundly, making you feel far more miserable the next morning.

52 Negative people bring you down. Surround yourself with miserable people, and it won't be long before you're moaning too. And that goes for bad relationships. They're a waste of time and energy, so get out now. Stuck with a rude, ungrateful boss? Find someone else who appreciates your skills.

53 Don't underestimate the power of your mind. If you've suffered a traumatic event, your mind will need extra energy to cope, which leaves your body in short supply. So be kind to your-self and take life easy until you're over the worst.

53 Candida is a yeast-like fungus which goes into overdrive when your body's good bacteria is attacked (the contraceptive pill and antibiotics can do the damage). Symptoms include thrush, IBS, bloating, constipation, diarrhea, and serious fatigue. If your energy levels are low, you'll need an anti-fungal product to fight off the fungus. A low-yeast, low-sugar diet will also help, as fungus feeds on these foods. Cut out all sugar and alcohol, and eat only fresh fruit in the morning. Resist bread, pasta, and pizza, and ditch the dairy products (eat soya and goat milk instead).

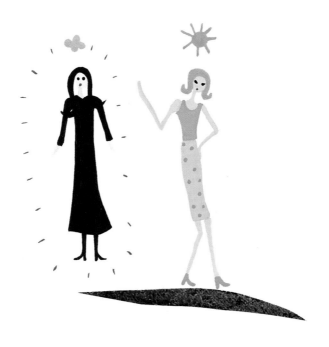

55 **It's not only sleep you're missing when you spend your nights in dark discos and bars.** It's fresh air too. Add the two together and guess who's going to feel bad the next day?

56 **Feeling low or depressed is your body's warning sign** that you have an energy crisis on your hands. Listen and learn from it.

57 **If you regularly suffer nodding head syndrome mid-afternoon,** chances are you're stuck in a centrally heated room. Any atmosphere with a low humidity level will make you feel tired and lethargic, and most offices are way too low. Place bowls of water near heat sources or invest in a humidifier to beat the post-lunch slump.

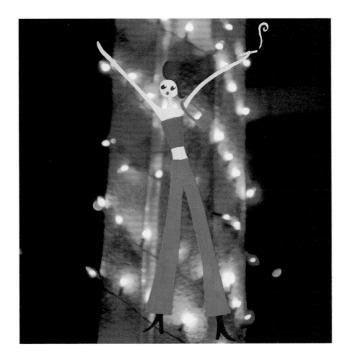

58 **Sore shoulders? Stiff neck?**
Muscular problems use up large amounts of energy, leaving little for the rest of your body to make it through the day. Take a break, stretch, treat yourself to a massage, visit an osteopath or chiropractor. Your body will thank you for it.

59 **If you suffer recurring digestive problems** (irritable bowel syndrome and bloating), low energy levels even after a good night's sleep, regular headaches, and even migraine attacks, chances are you may be sensitive to something you're putting in your mouth. While serious food allergies are downright dangerous, many more minor problems can be caused by a food intolerance. Migraine sufferers are often sensitive to cheese, chocolate, citrus fruit, and wine, while wheat can cause bloating and dairy products a stopped-up nose. To make matters more complicated, the very food that could be causing your problem may be the one you crave. Try cutting down on potentially unfriendly foods one at a time, or visit a dietician who'll be able to spot a food link much faster.

60 Negative thoughts drain your energy.

Instead of thinking the worst, or mulling over potential problems, visualize yourself in a positive setting and you gain energy from it. Don't think about all the complicated arrangements of going on vacation—imagine yourself already there. Visualize new opportunities such as a dream job, a new house, or a different environment. Your subconscious mind will respond to positive thoughts and act on them.

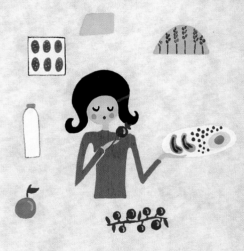

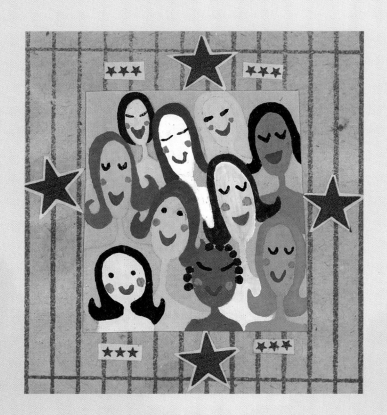

chapter 4

Energy friends

61 Natural light is an essential nutrient for your immune system. Make sure you spend some time outside every day and take off your sunglasses occasionally when it's not too bright so you get your full quota of sunlight. Light Therapy not only works to cure the symptoms of SAD. Putting differently colored light bulbs around your house can affect your energy levels too. If you want to feel full of vitality, sit under a bright orangy-red light.

Both yellow and pink light make you feel good, and blue bulbs will help you calm down at the end of a stressful day.

62 Twenty-first century technology can seriously sap your energy. Surround yourself with green plants both at home and in the office to help break down radiation coming from computers and televisions. The extra oxygen plants produce is an added energy saver.

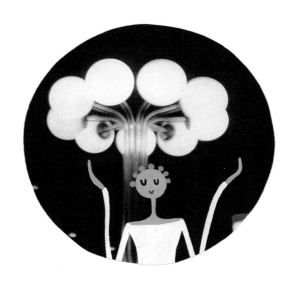

63 Doing something daring will give you an instant energy boost. Excite your senses by swimming in a dark or floodlit pool. Skinny dip for a guaranteed daredevil experience.

64 The sense of hearing is one of the earliest senses humans develop. Research has found that a newborn baby can recognize a piece of music played while they were in the womb. Music has been used in healing for thousands of years to energize and help people express their feelings. We instinctively use music to heal ourselves at home by listening to whatever makes us feel good. Avoid listening to continuous background music, and instead be aware of your emotional response to different songs and tunes—when you're tired or depressed, play upbeat music that makes you want to dance or brings back memories of happier times.

65 Find your energy hot-spot with a little do-it-yourself acupressure. Locate the sore point between your thumb and forefinger and press it firmly with your other hand. Continue pressing for a minute or two, and gradually release.

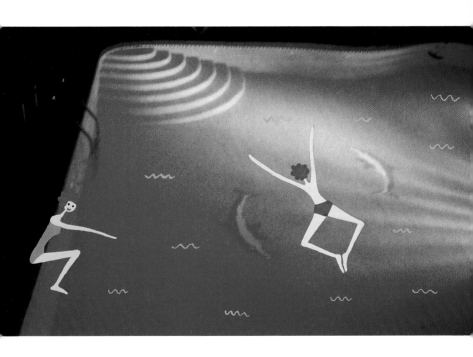

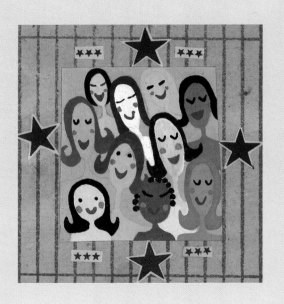

66 Start your mornings on the right note. Change your radio alarm to a soothing music station for a gentle wake-up call. There's nothing worse for your mood than being awakened by loud bells and buzzers.

67 Make time to have a good time. Ever wondered why children are always so full of beans? They're enjoying life.

68 **Energy-giving breath** = slow and deep from the abdomen. **Energy-sapping breath** = quick and shallow from the chest. **The best breath** = as you breathe in, your lungs expand to push out your stomach, and, as you breathe out, your stomach contracts to push out air. Lie on the floor and place one hand on your stomach to feel the movement. Consciously push out your stomach as you breathe in, and pull it in as you breathe out. Your body will naturally follow this pattern on the next breath. Keep this up for a few minutes until you become familiar with the feeling.

69 **Feel your body fading?** Give yourself a quick foot massage to stimulate all your pressure points. Kick off your shoes, wiggle your toes, and rotate your ankles. Then, starting at your heel, massage the whole of your foot in small circular movements. Bliss.

70 **This is strange, but true. Massaging your ears will make you feel more energetic.** Begin at the earlobe and use your finger and thumb to massage gently all the way up to the top of the ear. An instant mood improver— honest.

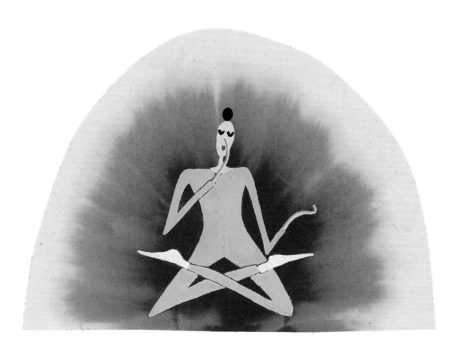

71 Most of us need between seven and nine hours of sleep to wake feeling refreshed, but research says most of us don't manage it. Apart from permanent tiredness, the result of too little sleep is headaches, bad moods, poor memory, and fuzzy sight. Here are some ways of getting a better night's sleep:

- *Avoid napping during the day, even if your eyes are closing and your head is nodding.*
- *Don't exercise after 9pm, as working out increases energy levels for several hours afterward.*
- *Don't go to bed until you feel tired. Tossing and turning is stressful, not soothing. If you're not asleep after an hour, get up and read. You want your bed to be associated with rest, not frustration.*
- *Take a warm bath 30 minutes before bedtime and add a sleep-inducing essential oil like lavender, chamomile, or sandalwood, mixed in well while the water is running.*
- *Break the nighttime hot chocolate habit. A cup of relaxing herbal tea will soothe you off to sleep far better. Try special nighttime infusions or chamomile tea.*
- *Warm milk has been proven to aid sleep. The protein in it is similar to one in the brain that regulates the body's sleep mechanism.*

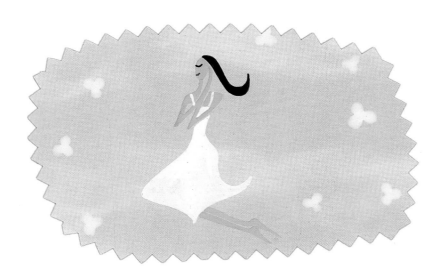

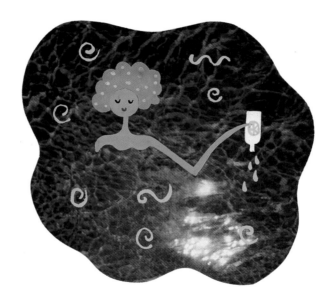

82

72 Erratic living will sap your energy. Try to keep your natural body clock consistent by going to bed and getting up at about the same time every day. Confusing your body's rhythms confuses your mind.

73 Get going in the morning with the help of a stimulating citrus oil in your shower or bath. A few drops of lemon or grapefruit will do the trick. Drop into your bath water, drip onto your shower floor, or add the oils to a sponge and rub them all over you, breathing deeply as you lather.

74 **Be open to new experiences.** Feel the fear, and enjoy it. Always dreamed of learning to waterski? Wanted to act since the school pantomime? New challenges leave your body and mind buzzing. So much better than yet another night spent in front of the TV.

75 **When you're feeling tired, add a few drops of peppermint oil to a tissue and inhale it frequently.** Or drip it onto a cotton handkerchief and lay the cloth over the top of your computer or a low-heat radiator. The aroma will fill your room and keep you alert throughout the day. Another way to scent your room is by dripping a little oil onto a light bulb. Turn on, and the heat will do the rest. If you need to concentrate for long periods, inhale rosemary oil as you work and it'll keep your mind focused.

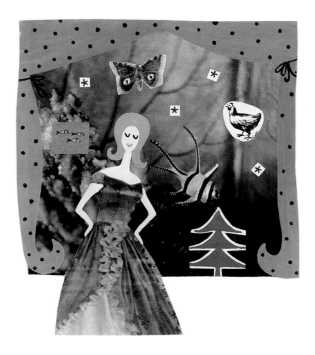

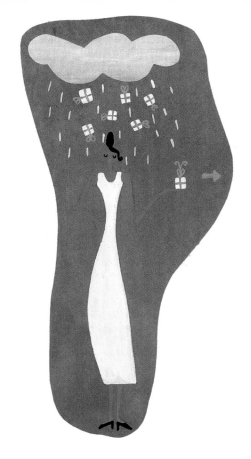

76 The law of karma states that what you give, you receive back in even larger quantities. So take time to give the gift of energy and happiness to others and they'll be only too pleased to return the favor.

77 **Low energy may mean an iron deficiency,** as iron helps red blood cells bring oxygen to the brain and muscles. Find it in meats, eggs, fish, green leafy vegetables, and dried fruit, or pop a vitamin pill containing iron to perk you up.

78 **Keep a mineral water spray in your bag or on your desk** and spritz your face when you're feeling bored or tired. A sure-fire way to wake up.

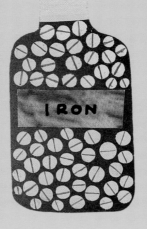

79 **Feng Shui practitioners say that cluttering up your home blocks the energy flow in your environment.** Even if you don't believe that a good clear out can redirect and realign energy, there's no denying that moving around a tidy house is much less exhausting than fighting your way through a mess every morning.

80 **Ever wondered why fast food burger bars are painted red, orange, and yellow?** Color is used every day to keep you moving and speed you up (so eating fast food means you don't occupy a seat for very long). You can use color to give yourself a shot of much-needed energy.

- *When you need a boost, focus on something red, yellow, or orange for a few minutes, so your mind can soak up the color's signals.*
- *If you're bored at work, surround yourself with orange to help bring you to life. Too much red interferes with decision making, and too much yellow affects concentration.*
- *Buy candles in a wide range of colors, and light the one that suits your mood. Orange lifts your spirits, pink wakes you up, and red sparks passion.*
- *Dull colors in winter can add to the depression of the long dark days. Switch to a bright color and your energy levels will lift immediately. If you're tired in the morning, wear something red.*

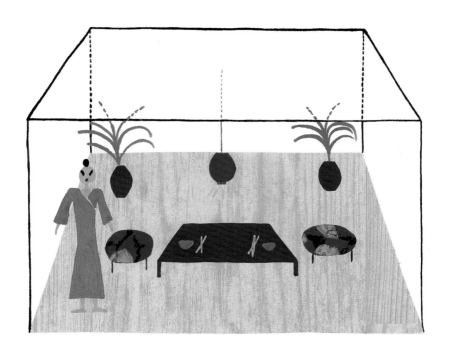

91

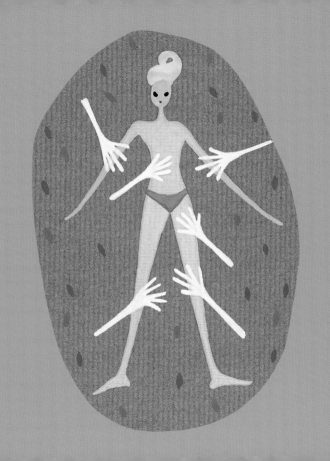

chapter 5

Energy treats

81 **Peppermint oil is a great pick-me-up.** Add six drops of oil to a bowl of warm water and soak your feet in it for ten minutes.

82 **Manipulate your own meridians for a do-it-yourself energy boost.** Feel around the bottom of your foot just under the pad that runs below your big toe and the start of your other toes and you should feel a W shape. Press deeply into the middle of it. Press with your thumb as you slowly breathe out. Repeat this movement for three to ten minutes to really feel the benefit, before doing the same on your other foot.

83 **Everyone knows a long luxurious bath leaves you lethargic.** Well, not necessarily. Water that is too hot increases your pulse rate, which drains your body of energy, but make the water around 95° F and you'll climb out raring to go.

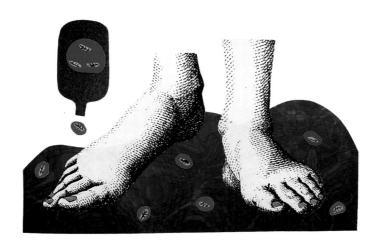

84 **For more hands-on healing at home, try a Shiatsu head massage to clear your mind.**

1. Using your fingertips, work from the front of your scalp to the back of your head using small circular movements.

2. Place one hand at the front of your head and one at the back and, moving both hands at the same time, work your fingers through your hair toward the top of your head using circular movements.

3. From the base of your neck, work up to the top of your head using circular movements. Apply firmer pressure to loosen tension.

85 **There's nothing like a massage to boost energy levels.** Most types of massage come from the East (even so-called Swedish massage) and are based on the idea of flowing energy. This built-up energy needs to be unblocked so your body can rebalance itself. The intimate contact also wakes up reflexes and feelings which activate your central nervous system. This floods your body with beneficial chemicals, boosting your immune system and promoting a feeling of deep relaxation. Add to this the release of muscle tension, and a massage is a must-have treat. Have one as often as you can afford it, or buy a book and learn to massage with a friend.

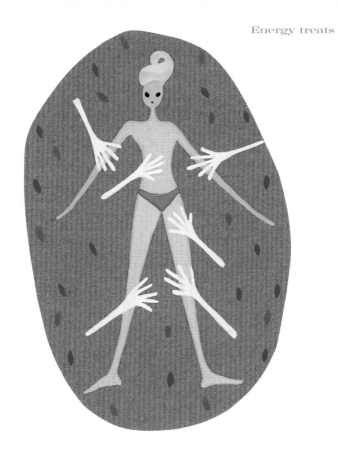

86 **Cold water will wake you up in the morning when you just feel like going back to bed.** If you're brave, a cold shower does the trick. Grit your teeth and turn the water to freezing for 30 seconds. Or give your body a boost before a busy evening by dipping your feet in cold water for 30 seconds at a time. Falling asleep on a night out? Hold an ice cube against your wrist pulse points, below your ears, or behind your knees for ten seconds.

87 **Ginseng has been used by the Chinese for years to boost energy.** This multi-talented herb works by stimulating the circulation, easing tension, and increasing stamina (ginseng is popular for treating a low libido). Ginseng can also help you cope with mental and physical stress, as it stimulates the release of energy-giving adrenaline into the bloodstream. It is available in capsules, as a herbal tea, and in energy drinks—for a useful midday boost.

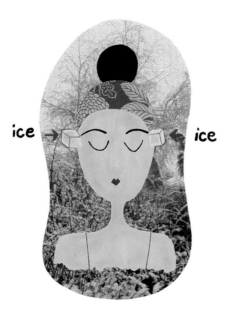

88 **Studies show that filling your surroundings with pleasant scents can improve your mental stamina and concentration.** For this, choose one of these energizing essential oils:

- *Black Pepper—makes you more alert*
- *Ginger—fights fatigue*
- *Bergamot—improves mood*
- *Lemon—keeps your focused and relaxed*
- *Eucalyptus—lifts depression*
- *Cinnamon—wakes up a tired mind*
- *Orange—helps concentration*
- *Ylang Ylang—works as an aphrodisiac.*

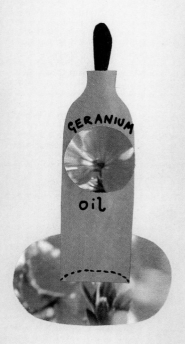

89 **Ancient Oriental medicine believes your energy (known as** *chi*) **flows along your meridians (energy pathways) inside your body.** When these paths are blocked, your energy cannot flow freely. Treatments aim to stimulate the flow of energy by removing the blocks, and you can expect to finish one feeling full of energy yet pleasantly relaxed. Here's what's on offer:

Shiatsu (Japanese massage)—you lie on a mat while the practitioner applies pressure to particular points on your meridians with his thumbs, fingers, and palms, and sometimes even his elbows, knees, and feet.

Reflexology—points on the hands and feet that correspond with internal organs are stimulated with the fingers and thumbs.

Acupuncture—very fine needles are applied to stimulate specific points.

Acupressure—similar to shiatsu, but only the fingers and thumbs are used.

90 **Zero balancing was developed in the 1970s,** the inspiration behind which was acupuncture, osteopathy and chiropractics. It aims to soothe and balance your physical and mental energies. The idea is that trauma can affect our subtle energy circulation, and zero balancing helps ease the flow. A practitioner will manipulate your whole body, moving and stretching it bone-deep, which may also release emotional stress.

91 **Fans of flotation describe it as the deepest rest they've ever known.** The feeling of total weightlessness frees the brain and body from gravity, which releases vast amounts of energy and brain power. In a flotation tank, there are also no outside distractions so you can relax deeply and focus on your body. One hour of floating in the tank is said to have the restorative effect of four hours of sleep, so it's not surprising you emerge with more energy.

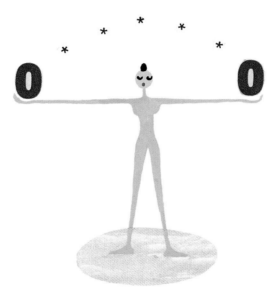

92 **The Amazonian Indians got their kicks from guarana,** a mild stimulant containing caffeine, theophylline, and tannin (all found in a cup of tea). One gram contains slightly less caffeine than a weak cup of black tea, but converts say it gives a much longer and better buzz. Chew guarana gum when you need to pep up your performance. Natural energizers include aloe vera juice, kelp, and co-enzyme Q10, which all boost your body in a healthy way.

Guaraná

93 **A glass of wheatgrass juice works as a shot of energy,** especially if you drink it straight from the blender so the active ingredients can shoot straight into your bloodstream. Find wheatgrass at juice bars and health food shops everywhere.

94 **A poor diet can block your body with toxic waste,** draining toxins into your bloodstream. Fans of colonic irrigation believe that flushing your colon with many liters of water will dislodge the debris. This may not sound much of a treat, but devotees report a serious energy boost afterward.

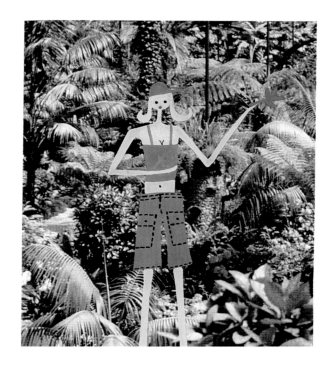

95 **Falling asleep when you should be concentrating?** Rush off to the bathroom and splash your face with cool water. Just make sure you're wearing waterproof mascara!

96 **Your body's not the only thing that gets tired.** Your mind needs a rest too. Just as muscles repair and strengthen when you take a break from exercise, so your mind must relax so that it may return to work refreshed. Get to know your own attention span and then take a guilt-free break to do something no more taxing then filing your nails. Developing your own personal work style will get the most out of your mind.

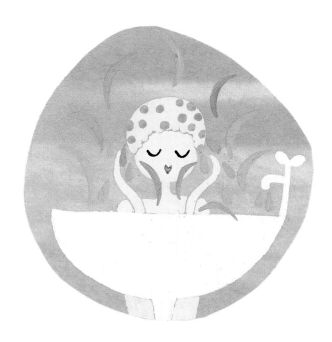

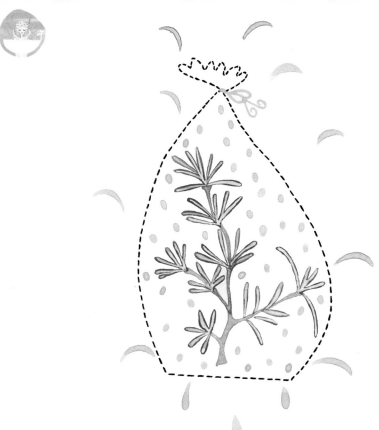

97 **Scrubbing your skin in the bath or shower will boost your blood circulation and energize your whole body.** Fill a small muslin bag with oatmeal and a sprig of rosemary and gently rub it all over your body, starting from the feet and working upward.

98 **Get going with ginger.** Grate a small handful of fresh ginger and squeeze the liquid into a bowl of hot water. Then dip a small hand towel into the mixture, wring it out, and hold on your lower back. This energy-boosting compress improves circulation and also soothes a sore back (a common energy-sapper).

99 Meditation slows down your body and mind so they can recharge their batteries. When you meditate, your heart rate decreases, your blood pressure falls, and your breathing becomes much slower. Just twenty minutes of meditation adds up to a mini-shutdown, which fans say is worth an hour's sleep. No wonder you feel so energized at the end. Try this do-it-yourself technique. Choose a quiet spot where you won't be interrupted and turn off the lights. Sit comfortably and imagine each part of your body relaxing, starting with your scalp and working downward to your toes. Now concentrate on a single neutral thought, such as a color, and focus on breathing deeply. Whenever a thought breaks through the calm, just let it go. After 20 minutes, slowly open your eyes and sit quietly for a short while before standing up.

100 Under pressure? Try this quick relaxation technique. You'll feel calmer instantly and have more energy to deal with what's worrying you. Take in a deep breath and tense all your muscles. Hold this pose for ten seconds and then release it on a big exhalation. Repeat this for a few times, breathing normally between exercises.

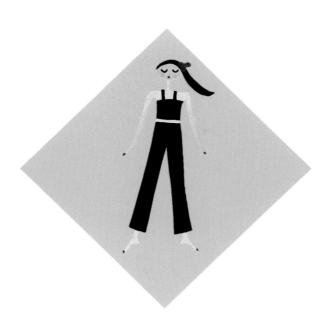

Copyright © MQ Publications Ltd 2002

Text © Liz Wilde 2002
Illustrations © Carol Morley 2002
Interior Design: Philippa Jarvis
Series Editor: Kate John

Time Warner Books are published by
Time Warner Trade Publishing
1271 Ave. of the Americas
New York, NY 10020

Visit our Web site at www.twbookmark.com

 An AOL Time Warner Company

Printed in China
First printing: 10 9 8 7 6 5 4 3 2 1

Library of Congress Control Number: 2001097176

ISBN: 1-931722-05-6